MW01235804

My War on
AGING

MOVING THROUGH LIFE

My War on
AGING

MOVING THROUGH LIFE

NANCY K. BURNHAM

This book is not intended as a substitute for the medical advice of physicians. The reader should regularly consult a physician in matters relating to his/her health and particularly with respect to any symptoms that may require diagnosis or medical attention.

Publishing, composition, and design managed by Niche Pressworks
http://nichepressworks.com

ISBN Print: 978-1-946533-07-4
ISBN Digital: 978-1-946533-08-1

Dedication

This book is dedicated to my children, my grandsons, and everyone who ever doubted they could control their health or wanted to do more but did not know how.

Acknowledgements

My thanks to Dr. Robert Pruni, my personal trainer and chiropractor for five years who pushed me to my brink on more than one occasion.

My gratitude to Tina Smith, friend extraordinaire, who kept telling me God would provide all that I needed and to never give up. Her spiritual counseling was incredible.

To Todd Rogers Terry, friend, actor, and personal trainer, who taught me much about weight lifting and humanity—my life is better for having known you. I am forever grateful.

Table of Contents

Foreword

Having been in practice for over three decades and seeing and treating pain and dis-ease in its many forms one thing has always prevailed. Health and wellbeing begins from within. Our bodies are amazing miracles of nature with a preprogrammed will to survive. All too often I have seen patients whose chosen path in life has taken them down what seems to be "the path of no return" causing them to have to battle with ailments, many of which are nothing but an outcome of a chosen lifestyle. Unfortunately in today's society the average person will seek the resolution to these health challenges from medication and even surgery. That is not to say that medicine and good professional healthcare is not a necessity, but rather that medicine and good professional healthcare is not a necessity, but rather that *in so many instances it is not the true solution to the cause of what ails us.*

Nancy's book is a heartwarming story of personal triumph. A tale of how, no matter at what point in life, it is never too late to take charge of our lives. To realize that at the end it is us who hold the true key to our health and wellbeing. In this book, she shares her true experience of how a state of desperation, pain and disease became the driving force behind the challenging, and at times seemingly impossible decision of taking the steps to take control of one's life, health and destiny. It is a story that all too often has remained untold.

If you are reading this, congratulate yourself as you may be at the start of this very path as all paths in life begin with "the first step". The fact that you have reached this point by reading these words means that YOU, too, have already taken that step. Read her story of pain, desperation, perseverance and ultimate triumph in her journey and let it be a life lesson that could guide and inspire you.

Dr. Hamid Sadri, DC, CCSP, ICCSP, CSCS, CES, PES

Preface

When I was a senior in high school, my mother worked as a nurse in the emergency room of the local hospital. On holidays my family would go to the hospital to spend a little time with her and experience some of the trauma she dealt with on a regular basis. When she had a meal break we went to the cafeteria to enjoy a meal with her. I often said I would someday write a book about the many personalities she encountered during her career there.

When I retired from the federal judicial system I considered writing a book about my life as I struggled being a divorced single mother working full time, attending college at night, and raising two children. All the while both my parents were aging and I could see role reversal on the horizon. There never seemed to be time to write.

Years passed. Life continued to happen and I tried to adapt. Then, one day, the urge to write returned but at that time I was unsure what to write or how to express what I felt.

After I survived my first year of personal training which defied my body's aging processes and rejuvenated my life, I determined now was the time to get serious about putting words on paper. It was time to explain the journey that has changed me forever. Though the urge to write started some time ago, my knowledge of and insights into how my body moved continued to grow exponentially. My perspective on life evolved into something quite different than it had been in the past. So now I write to share with you this miraculous war I waged on aging.

I believe that to whom much is given much is required. I have been given an opportunity to help others by sharing my story and my talents to teach. It is our individual responsibility to keep our body in the best condition possible as it adapts to metabolic and muscular changes.

Albert Einstein said, "Strive not to be a success but rather to be of value." The purpose of this book is to plant the seed in your heart and mind that *you have the power and strength to control your health and aging process.*

Take control now to enjoy your future. It is never too late!

Introduction

As a child I loved school. I enjoyed learning and I enjoyed my teachers—most of the time. What I did not like about school were some of my classmates because of the things they said and did to me. "Fatty, fatty, two by four, can't get in the bathroom door, so she did it on the floor." I heard the chant many times in my years of grammar school.

My parents were clueless about the teasing and turned a deaf ear to anyone thinking I was anything but "wholesome." The sound of that word makes me shiver with shame even now. It was a very different era. We felt good about the food on our table. No one ever spoke about being "fat," it was always "healthy," "full-figured," or "wholesome."

Society places labels on us as we age. Our body changes and we are told from age forty onward, "at your age…." Doctors, news publications, our society's values, have adopted the theme that aging equals less ability, less physical strength, and less mental and emotional ability. Rarely do we find a medical professional that tells us to eat plenty of vegetables, lift weights for muscle retention and good bone strength, and get good solid sleep. That would take more time than writing a prescription to take a pill.

When I went back to school (college) at thirty-five, recently divorced and raising two children alone, my perspective, of course, was quite different than that of an adolescent. Yes, I still enjoyed learning, sometimes I liked my instructors, but I did not spend much time with the others in my classes because I was working full-time and raising a family. It was all about survival. I lived and worked in a man's world and struggled to make a good living for the children, and, if possible, a retirement income.

Oh, the power of 20/20 hindsight. If only we knew then what we know now, how different our world would/*could* be.

Our body clock keeps ticking. Our metabolism changes. Our wants and needs never seem to be met and we succumb to society's dictates. And most of us move to the beat of society's drummer that sets our ebb and flow of life. *We feel but cannot see* the cumulative internal changes occurring.

My generation was not taught to ask the hard questions. We were not taught to question the doctor; What is the purpose of this medication? Why do we need that surgery? What will the long-term effects be? What are the possible side effects? What else might I do to stop this nagging pain? I lifted something the wrong way—will you teach me the right way? When the scale tipped too far no one said I needed to change the carbohydrates or fat in my diet. What is the difference between a carbohydrate and a protein anyway? Why should I care? But then, my ancestors died young so it was assumed I would too.

I was taught that an ounce of prevention is worth a pound of cure, but was not told to apply that to my ongoing health journey.

Where along life's road did I/we/you give all the power to others to dictate our future health and longevity? I am really not sure, but I can tell you for certain that *it is never too late to change your life. Take this journey with me as I share with you what I learned while moving through life in my sixties.*

My mantra became I CAN DO THIS and YOU can too.

YOU have the power.

Chapter I
LIFE HAPPENS -
THE ODDS ARE AGAINST ME

Proceed as if success is inevitable.
—Unknown

I pulled up in the parking lot and sat there checking my watch. *What was I doing?* What was going to happen to me in this place? I felt so vulnerable, so stupid, so, so, afraid. So much that was unknown was ahead of me. My mind just could not imagine how terrible I would look walking on a treadmill. My eyes would not leave the images behind the wall of windows. Just look at all those people with headphones. Sweat was rolling down their faces, yet they looked content.

No, I would not look at the people or the machines. I would just wait and find out for myself. "I must be jumping to conclusions because I am feeling insecure," I told myself. I had live or die concerns. It was 2008 and those other people didn't care about my issues. Surely they had their own to be concerned about and mine would make no difference to them. They didn't care what I looked like, or what equipment I used, or how slowly I walked, or what I wore to hide my body. No, they had their own reasons to be there. Surely they would not notice me.

So, with difficulty, imagining my worst fears come true, I stepped out of the car, made my way to the door and walked into the gym. The clerk at the desk asked me to wait; so I did. She came back almost instantly and said Dr. Pruni, my personal trainer, would be with me in a few minutes. I stood there listening to the clank of the weight machines, the whirr of the stationary bikes, and the whop, whop of the elliptical machines trying to hide just how scared I really was. And then he appeared.

Dr. Pruni was all business. It was clear from his sculpted body that he had trained for years. There was no way that I could know what he had in mind for me. He was older than the other trainers moving around in the background. He said nothing about his credentials—just studied my membership form. My health issues were listed: High cholesterol, high blood pressure, two prolapsed heart valves, asthma/COPD, anxiety, depression, chronic pain from arthritis, and, of course, excess weight. At the age of sixty-one, I had five prescription medications and a lot of pain. There were questions about my diet—which I thought was pretty good—but obviously, it was not and had not been for a while. He was busy writing notes as he spoke. I knew he was speaking but somehow had difficulty understanding everything. But I did hear the words, "I can help but it will take a while."

Help. That was what I had come here for. It was a four-letter word that spoke volumes to my pain. Yes, I could believe it would take "a while" but just how long was that in emotional time as opposed to clock and calendar time? I was about to find out the real cost of changing my life.

We established a schedule; three mornings a week. I was to come fifteen minutes early and warm-up (whatever that meant), then we would work thirty minutes and I would do a fifteen-minute cool down (whatever that meant). If possible, I was to come in at least two additional days a week and follow the same routine of warm-up, workout, cool down. We had to start changing my metabolic rate. What? It was a lot to take in for a thirty-minute session. I knew when to come back and I would be there. After all, he had said he would help and I had put my money and my body on the line here.

When I was born in 1947, technology at that time had no way to know which genes were being passed along from our parents or grandparents. As we travel along life's road some things just show up now and again. Most often we help them show up. But then, we find surprises come to join the party in our body; maybe allergies or high blood pressure. Sometimes something worse develops.

The medical system seems to think that age is directly related to physical illness. But, *it ain't necessarily so. Research has found exercise/ physical activity can lessen some chronic illnesses.*

My mother passed away when I was forty-one. It took several years for her to receive an accurate diagnosis of Addison's disease. Wasn't it enough that she had suffered from allergies to a number of foods and animals, been plagued with back pain, and ultimately become allergic to the sun? That was enough. But for her children to carry the fear of a possible terminal illness should be changed IF it can be changed.

At age forty-nine, I was diagnosed with osteoarthritis in both hands and both feet. Not good. Sure, I was working sixty hours a week while going to college at night for several years, but whoa, that arthritis stuff is serious. It's not easy to type with swollen fingers or write essays with your hand and arm in a brace. Taking Aleve at intervals during the day just to keep moving resulted in stomach problems. Many adults share this tragedy.

At fifty-four, leaving home for work on a Friday morning, I passed out as I started to lock the stairwell door. I came to as my body tumbled down the steps, striking my head repeatedly as I continued to tumble to the concrete floor. Subsequently, I suffered a concussion and damaged the rotator cuff on my left shoulder. Life kept moving along day after day after day. I cared for others and did my job as best I could. The injured shoulder froze in place and eventually required six months of physical therapy to recover full use.

My father occasionally had pneumonia. Then came the heart attack at age seventy that required double bypass surgery. I thought all that was enough to deal with as a forecast for my "Golden Years." Crazy me! I was in for a surprise—or four or five or six!

At age fifty-eight, I was forced to take a look at my future and it was not good. Over a nine-month period, I was surprised by bad-news-times-six. Physician-ordered testing at Emory confirmed I had: (1) asthma on the scale of low-level COPD; (2) residual fluid in my lungs; (3) two prolapsing heart valves; (4) anxiety; (5) major depressive disorder; and (6) high cholesterol. Boom!

The osteoarthritis pain was already a daily companion. Adventures with Morton's Neuroma, bunions, and foot surgery were added to my list of ongoing health experiences. Low back pain was a regular visitor as well. I really did not know what I did not know about my health. I adapted to survive each day.

As I continued to prepare for retirement at sixty, the flashbacks began; I could see my mother and my father sitting at the kitchen table performing their morning routine of first one prescription pill, then another, then another. Routine refilling of prescriptions and filling the blocks on the calendar with multiple ongoing doctor appointments occupied most of their time.

What was my future? What was going on with me that I did not know? How would I know if anything else changed?

The odds were against me. But what the universe did not know was I was mad as hell with the health system, with doctors in general, with the medical community's assumptions about aging, with society's labeling of "seniors," and all the other concepts about getting old.

Yes, I was mad as hell and I would not stand for it. This is my life and I am in control. So I did the only thing I knew to do. "Diet and exercise," the doctors say. Well, here I come—alone, afraid, and feeling really stupid. Look out World, cause you are in for a fight!

Chapter 2

PAIN

Most people spend more time and energy going around problems than in trying to solve them.
— Henry Ford

It continued day and night; pain in the shoulder, pain in the hands, pain in the lower back, pain in the knee, and sciatic pain. What part of this was "golden"? My hands were so swollen that I could not button my clothes. Each time I tried to bend my first finger, the pain was excruciating. How could I possibly work this way if I can't dress myself? Osteoarthritis had taken a large toll on my hands, my feet and my spine but I did not know how debilitating it would ultimately become.

Some years earlier during a visit to the emergency room with my significant other (who was in extreme pain and trying to be brave), the doctor sensed his condition and remarked, "Being in pain serves no *good* purpose." But pain is a warning signal from our body. Isn't that a good thing?

Many millions of us are in pain—all levels of pain—every day. In some cases, we do not know the root cause of the pain. In most circumstances, we continue to treat pain, even if we know the root cause because we become complacent, believing that taking a pill will make it go *away or* become bearable. No matter if it is osteoarthritis, tendonitis, headache, knee, or stomach pain, we blindly take pain medications and keep going. Why? It serves no good purpose, both literally and figuratively to do this. We try not to think about the pain, but our body is speaking to us, sending a message, *"Something is not right."*

We do not want to seem impaired by our pain. We do not want to be limited in our mobility or our ability to sit comfortably in a chair. Even worse, we do not want the pain to disrupt our mental or emotional stability. But we know it can and ultimately will. What can we wear to conceal the swelling in the knee or leg that aches so deeply down to the bone? How do we manage to retain focus during the day?

My pain was there every morning, every night, over and over. Day after day I functioned with pain to the extent I was taking five Aleve every day. Pain. Sharp pain that seared my brain. Dull, deep, aching pain that pierces the bone. *Why is it here and what does it have to teach me?* Have you ever asked these questions? Without questions, we have no answers and without answers, we do not know *how to treat the pain.* Are we afraid to ask because we don't really want to know? Or do we not ask because we know the doctor will not hear us?

We can understand temporary traumatic pain because the cause is evident and logical. Pain with a broken bone or torn muscle can be tolerated and treated because we know it will eventually end. But why, oh why, do we tolerate or pharmaceutically treat long-term pain without knowing and understanding the cause? What belief system told us this is ok? What physician advocates this without investigating the cause? How does the medical community continue to survive without treating patients with corrective information?

Moreover, what are those pain medications doing to your body? Your stomach and liver will really know the difference. Too much cortisone weakens your cell structure. Too much aspirin can cause serious stomach problems.

The body speaks to us but it is *our* responsibility to listen and take corrective action. When did we give that responsibility to someone else? There are answers but we must first ask the questions.

Each morning as I opened my eyes I took an inventory of my body's aches and pains. As a beginning student of physical training, it was necessary for me to communicate to my trainer exactly what I was feeling and experiencing physically. It was the trainer's responsibility to know how to use that information.

A good trainer sees the look in your eyes, the tightening of your jaw when you grit your teeth, the sweat on your face, the deep breaths you take, or that you are holding your breath. A good trainer is truly a trained observer of your body. If your knee hurts, you walk differently. If your shoulder hurts, you favor it by decreased range of motion. If your hip hurts, you most likely will limp. These pains cannot stay hidden when the body is moving. Make no mistake about one thing— the body was made *to move*.

So how long have you had these pains and how badly do you want to rid yourself of them? Are you willing to trust someone else with the task of guiding you through the "tough" part or are you just afraid to try? Why?

A better question yet is, do you want to avoid the possibility of having pain? Aristotle said, "education is the best provision for the journey to old age." Take the time to educate yourself about the cause of your pain and you will never regret it. This is a journey you are on and it behooves us all to plan that journey well.

Do you not trust yourself enough? Do you not truly *believe* there is a way to stop the pain that does not include prescription medication? There are, of course, exceptions to the rule. Common sense dictates that we can, however, control more than we admit. What are you willing to admit about your pain?

For too long we habitually settle for "take two aspirin and call me in the morning." This is not an answer. It is a postponement of healing.

I have labeled my right knee as my "old" knee and my left knee as my "surgery" knee. They both pop, crack, and make noise from time to time but the left one more so because I have very little medial meniscus.

My left knee was first to speak to me when it completely stopped moving in December 2005. I was absolutely clueless about knee structure except I had heard "old" people complain about knee aches. My "anatomical aging" lesson was about to begin.

As you may know, orthopedic remedies have come a long way since then. The condition I was experiencing is known as Patella Femoral Syndrome, also known as Runner's Knee, and is quite common in the aging process. I was only fifty-eight. By the time it flared up again at sixty-two, I was in the midst of my newly found exercise regime. This time there was no six-week period of physical therapy. Instead, I received a shot of synthetic joint fluid, rested the knee from strenuous exercises such as lunges and deep squats for about two weeks and I was good as new for the next eighteen months.

As time passed I learned the "three-day rule" for pain. This was immensely helpful for me and I have passed it along to all of my clients. Following rigorous exercise for a particular part of the body, we are likely to have soreness in muscles that have not been used frequently. Ladies, have you washed windows lately? Men, were you tossing that football or shooting hoops with the kids all afternoon and woke up the next morning to shoulder aches and pains? If so, you just found a weak spot in your back and shoulders.

Each time my trainer taught me an exercise (that ultimately caused pain for a day or two afterward), I went home to research the anatomical area. To my surprise, most often the pain was not from a single muscle but from two or three. Whoever heard of such nonsense as muscles working together? My light bulb moments just kept coming. Not only were the muscles in groups but they moved in multiple directions together. WOW!

Day one after exercise it is normal to have some mild aches and, possibly, pain. Use ice to decrease the inflammation. *If* you have pain at the same level or worse on day two, then continue the ice use and pamper the affected area. *If* on day three the pain has not lessened, feel free to consult a physician or just not exercise the area for a few days. RICE is the common acronym for Rest, Ice, Compression, and Elevation. Most often this is used with sprained ankles but is also good for other soreness and/or muscular injuries.

Always be mindful of the onset of a very sharp pain which could indicate an injury to the muscles or supporting structure.

Pain triggers other reactions in our bodies that we may not see. We have swelling and redness with simple thorn pricks but we can also have swelling and tenderness from muscle activity. These are visible signs that other reactions are taking place in our body. This is inflammation.

Inflammation is a message, an indicator, that something else is going on and needs our attention. It is our body speaking to us asking for help. Inflammation has far-reaching reactions. It raises our cholesterol levels. It can cause pain in our joints.

Although we generally think of cholesterol as "bad," it also serves other purposes within our bodies. There is much more activity in the body than meets the eye. Chain reactions are happening all the time, they are just not visible until the worst happens.

Pain is only one of the methods our body uses to speak to us but it is the one most often noticed. Pain should never be ignored.

Chapter 3
BELIEVE YOU CAN

From Alice in Wonderland
"There is no use trying," said Alice; "one can't believe impossible things." "I dare say you haven't had much practice," said the Queen. "When I was your age, I always did it for half an hour a day. Why, sometimes I've believed as many as six impossible things before breakfast."
—Lewis Carroll

For some unknown reason, I never read <u>Alice in Wonderland</u> when I was a child. I knew the premise of the story. In the movie I saw Alice fell down the rabbit hole and had an adventure, in a dream that included some crazy characters. She had adventures that gave her new perceptions of life. I did not know there would be several good messages in the story.

Some years ago, while in a bookshop, I saw a quote from the story that intrigued me. "There is no use trying," said Alice; "one can't imagine impossible things."

Needless to say, I just had to watch the movie to see where this fit in. Alice was talking with the White Queen (the good queen). Alice felt it impossible to imagine her ability to fight the Jabberwock (dragon) to end the rule of the Red Queen (bad queen) and fear in the kingdom.

"I daresay you haven't had much practice," said the Queen. "When I was your age, I always did it for half an hour a day. Why, sometimes I've believed as many as six impossible things before breakfast."

Do you still use your imagination? Wikipedia defines imagination as "...the process of forming new images in the mind that have not been previously experienced, or at least only partially or in different combinations." Try now to recall the last time you said, "I wish," or "I'm not able to do . . . ," or "I can't do that." We are never too old to use our imagination to benefit our health.

There is a definite mind-body connection.

When we are unable to use our imagination we are selling ourselves short of receiving possible miracles. We are not experiencing life in its fullest. Keep in mind that our brain directs our body not the reverse. Train you brain to teach your body how to move and heal.

Belief in our imagination and our strengths and abilities is tied to health recovery. As adults, we have beliefs about life's structures and routines. It is so easy to fall into someone else's belief about us. Why? Where is your imagination and courage?

Albert Einstein said, "Imagination is more important than knowledge. For knowledge is limited to all we now know and understand, while imagination embraces the entire world and all there ever will be to know and understand."

Wow, what possibilities we have! As for my exercise adventures, on many days I found it difficult to believe in my abilities. While learning new moves with three elements of form; the placement of the feet, engaging the core, using the back instead of the shoulders, I sometimes had to step back, clear my mind and try again. "Too much!" my mind would scream. Then we would try it again. This time it was a little better. The third try was usually the best.

One day amidst my challenges, I began to mutter ever so quietly to myself, "I can do this." That didn't seem very convincing. Then it came again and I muttered, "I can do THIS." By then I was really ready to believe in me and I said, "I CAN do this." In that moment it did not matter to me who was there watching or listening. It only mattered that I try with every ounce of my imagination because my life depended on it.

I did not know at that time how much progress I would make or what would happen to me along the way. If I could believe that my "imagination embraces the entire world and all there ever will be to know and understand," then I could do anything I set my mind to.

It meant: I could make my breath come easier when I ran.

It meant that my heart rate would be steady as I made one more lap around the parking lot.

It meant each time I achieved a victory, however small, the depression and anxiety took a day off.

It meant I could carry my groceries up the steps without stopping to catch my breath.

It meant I could play touch football with my grandson. It mean that I could think more clearly and smile more often.

It meant I could live a longer, happier life.

Chapter 4
THE ORDER OF THINGS

There is nothing more difficult to take in hand, more perilous to conduct, or more uncertain in its success than to take the lead in the introduction of a new order of things.
–Niccolo Machiavelli, 1532

The year 1532 was a very long time ago, but it seems some folks back then did not like change any more than some people I know today. Some things never seem to change. But we know all too well that change is sometimes necessary. Likewise, there is good in some matters, "If it ain't broke, don't fix it."

Is your health "broken?" Does it need "fixing?" Do you want to get ahead of the chronological and biological changes that occur?

This old dog can learn new tricks, but it takes time. Slowly I began to learn the order of things. It was simple in some ways but more challenging in other ways because I did not understand the body yet.

I went to the gym to work with Dr. Pruni on Monday, Wednesday, and Friday each week. On the other weekdays, I went in and did cardio for at least thirty minutes. For me to really get myself into this exercise thing I had to understand what was going on.

I was showing up five days a week and it was time to really get down to business. Who was making this decision—my heart or my head? The truth was it was neither of those.

The truth was that I wanted to know I would and could live without the pain, the embarrassment, the awkwardness, and suffering my mother had endured. It took years to get an accurate diagnosis of Addison's disease. She alternated her pain meds to avoid addiction. She worked as long as she could, caring for others though tired and suffering in silence. No, I did not want my mother's frailty and early death.

It was true that I had neglected my own health to care for others, to earn my retirement, and to help my children on the road to their future. Now it was time to try and right the wrongs I had done to my physical and mental health. Now it was time to put my nose to the grindstone and get the job done—one day at the time, one hour at the time.

A week has seven days—seven opportunities to take one hour out of twenty-four to make that effort. How hard could that be? Really, how hard? Every possible excuse came to mind, but they were just that, excuses, not valid reasons.

When we know what to expect, our mind can adapt—maybe. When we don't know what to expect (how really, really, hard it will be), it seems a bit easier. The bottom line is you are either going to do it or you're not.

Half-ass won't cut it. Half-ass only shows you really don't care enough or want it bad enough. Sixty-one is not the usual age in life to make difficult decisions about changing your life. But that was where I was and there was no turning back, no more waking up every day with pain, no taking prescription medications that were doing terrible things to my body.

I WILL CHANGE THE ORDER OF MY LIFE. I ACCEPT THAT IT WILL BE DIFFICULT AT TIMES, BUT I WILL DO THIS.

In my mind each day I began to build a framework of movements corresponding to various muscles of the body. Warm-up was fifteen minutes before my thirty-minute full workout (most days), followed by a fifteen-minute cool down. The thirty-minute session was tough to learn. That is until I began to come out of pain.

> Mondays were shoulders, triceps, and abdominals.
> Wednesdays were legs, biceps, and abdominals.
> Fridays were chest, back, and abdominals.

There were seated shoulder presses with dumbbells, front raises, side lateral raises, shoulder shrugs, triceps kickbacks, French presses, triceps pushdown, rope extensions, closed grip bench press, dips, squats, leg presses, leg curls, leg lunges, toe raises, hack squats, stiff-legged deadlifts, bicep curls, hammer curls, concentration curls, preacher curls, bench presses, incline bench presses, dumbbell flies, seated rows, one arm rows, bent over row, lateral pull down, crunches, incline reverse crunch, hanging crunches, planks, side planks, wall balls, jump ropes, mountain climbers, and sit-ups, and any other functional training movement you could imagine.

These exercises were words I had never heard before. For the first few months I had to get specific instructions from Dr. Pruni because I did not know which movement went with which day or body parts. It was/is like putting a puzzle together.

Some days I cried the entire time as I went from machine to machine. But I was moving; lifting the weight or pulling the weight. I was changing my chemistry, but it was difficult. Showing up is the first step. It slowly began to get better. No, I did not say it got easier because it took a long time for it to get easier to make the moves. Showing up became easier.

I tried whatever he threw at me. Success was not always the result, but at least I tried. I hung from a bar, I did incline sit-ups, and I threw weighted balls against the building. Some days were just hard, but I showed up.

Several occasions during my workouts stand out in my mind. Several months into my training I went to the dip machine, which was truly my nemesis (and still is). I would plead with Doc not to make me do dips, but of course, there was no such possibility.

I stepped up and took my position, hung my head in desperation and started moving. When we stopped for a short rest a lady came up to me on my left and commented, "You have no idea how much you inspire me and others here in the gym. You come in every day and work so hard but don't give up. I just wanted you to know how you inspire me to do more."

I just stood there with my empty mind and blank face, not knowing what to say. Doc came to my rescue and thanked her for me. All I could think was that people were watching me. That would never do. Who was I to be watched and admired?

One day as I was trying to do squats on the BOSU™ ball my left foot turned out and I heard an awful "snap" sound, followed by excruciating pain. Heads turned. Machines stopped. Doc said he thought I had broken my ankle. I agreed and we moved on to another exercise. After the workout, we went to his office for an x-ray and confirmed the ligament had snapped the bone. The next day I saw the orthopedist and he put me in a not-so-lovely plastic boot to wear for several weeks.

Any ordinary "old lady" would not go back to the gym for a few days. But no, that did not stop me from training. The treadmill was not so easy to maneuver so I stuck to the elliptical for my warm-ups. Whatever the moves of the day were, we went through them the best that I could. Folks looked at me like I was the craziest person in the building. And I most likely was. I might represent a few adjectives about my personality but "quitter" was not one of them.

That was in late September 2010—about eighteen months after I began my training.

Later that year, as the weights on my lifts increased, the "guys" began to take notice. Sometimes I wondered if they thought about their mother possibly being in my shoes. Thanks to the revealing wall of mirrors, I was able to quickly glance over and see who was watching. Doc pulled two benches close to each other, then he took the plank position with hands on one bench and feet on the other and explained the leg and arm movements to make. My remark as I looked first at him and then at the benches was, "You want me to do what?"

Doc looked at me. I looked at him. The group of men working out looked at us both. Was the old lady really going to do it or not?

Fear, doubt, and anxiety all jumped into my head, each trying to make the most impact on my sanity. I stepped back, took a deep breath, tried to place my courage foremost in my mind. Planks on the floor was fine but planks twelve inches off the floor was a whole new notion for my brain to recognize. As I began to mumble

"I can do this. **I can do THIS. I CAN do this. I CAN DO THIS."**

And I did. And everyone watched. I had earned new respect from some of the guys in the heavy metal section. I could tell their surprise by the shocked facial expressions. Maybe it wasn't perfect, but at least I had done my best at the time.

I had learned a new order of things in my mind. I had learned to believe in me just a little more. But I still experienced moments of doubt, embarrassment, and panic.

My biggest challenges were yet to come.

Some months later Doc cut training sessions back to two days per week and it became necessary to adjust my training schedules and exercises. For me, this seemed like a big change in the now-comfortable order.

This made me more responsible for learning how and what to do on which days. By this time I was making a habit of regularly researching my aches, pains, broken bones, and sprained muscles. In late 2011 I started considering the idea of becoming a certified personal trainer.

Initially, the thought really scared me, but I knew that most older adults did not have trainers in the gym and did not know how to use the equipment correctly—or to their best advantage. When I was ready as a student, my teacher had appeared. Now it was time to give back.

It had been twelve years since I had last gone to school and taken exams. I never did well on exams. After much anxiety and some sleepless nights, I determined to try. I signed up with the American Council on Exercise and started my studies.

Little did I know what a big year 2012 was going to be.

In February of that year, I ran a 5K and took first place in my age bracket. Previously, in 2011, I had taken a third-place win.

Doc was pushing me pretty hard, but he kept encouraging me too. There was still anxiety in my mind when we would run laps in the parking lot, or he would have me do my workouts on the sidewalk outside the gym. I knew all those folks on the treadmills and bikes were watching me, just waiting for me to goof up and give up.

I never did. Sometimes they gave me a high five or shouted to me from the treadmill when I came back inside the gym.

By this time I had been off all five of my prescription medications for almost three years. Blood pressure was good. I had strengthened my heart valves as I had many other muscles.

My life had truly taken on a new order in exercise, in body recovery, and mental wellness. How far could I go? What more could I learn?

The best was yet to come. It was already happening, but I failed to recognize it at the time. Neuroplasticity, the ability of the brain to create new neural pathways, was already in progress. Proprioception was getting better every day. Arms and legs learned to move together. Soon the vertigo was almost nonexistent. My balance had improved tremendously.

You see, the mind sends messages to the muscles in our body to tell them what moves to make. During early development, these messages become automated as we learn to walk, run, jump, and hop. Each time we learn a new movement, or combination of moves, we are sending neuromuscular messages to our body.

However, if you don't use it, you lose it. The brain has to be activated just like everything else in our "movement" system.

The bottom line is that the brain tells the body what to do—the body does not tell the brain. That is the order of learning to exercise our body. If we think, believe and tell ourselves we can do something, *there is no reason not to try*.

It is not uncommon to find clients who cannot move their toes at will. When asked about this there seems to be no awareness of this inability. The Great Toe, as the big toe is termed, is crucial in the neural transmissions to our leg muscles. While this may sound a bit crazy, I ask the client to close their eyes, picture their Great Toe and think or talk to themselves out loud saying, "move toe." Quite to their surprise, the toe begins to move. This is an amazingly simple way to see the effectiveness of neuromuscular messages.

If this technique works with the toes, imagine how powerful it can be for other movements in our body. "Believe you can and you are halfway there," said Theodore Roosevelt.

Believe in the order of mind over matter and send those messages to your body.

Chapter 5
JUST BREATHE

Spirit has 50 times the strength and staying power
of brawn and muscle.
–Unknown

We have many four-letter words in the English vocabulary. Each one of them was created by us to express something. Fear is definitely a four-letter word we can be apprehensive about. Sometimes fear drives us to do bad things, and sometimes it drives us to do good things. Sometimes we freeze in fear doing nothing at all. But wait. Doing nothing is doing something. It says everything is ok, but I really am not happy with that. Ambivalence, complacency, and laziness can all be the result of unspoken fear.

As the new "mud runs" and CrossFit™ functional training began to move into the area, my workouts took on some new moves. High-Intensity Interval Training (HIIT) became the "fat-burning" workout for the fitness industry.

If there was one thing I had learned, *it was that it is necessary to make yourself vulnerable in the face of fear in order to learn to trust your instincts.* Ascertain what you have learned about life. With this in mind and my injuries in the past, I was encouraged to do the Warrior Dash, a 5K mud run with twelve obstacles.

It certainly must have been a day I was feeling brave when I signed up. If ever there was fear of something new this was it. I researched video from all over the United States to be sure I knew what was included. To do this would take all the courage I had gained and then some.

I knew about running a 5K because I had done three. What I had not done and had no way to practice, was obstacles. How was I to prepare without ropes for rope climbs, cargo nets to practice climbing on, tires to run through or fences to climb?

First I started practicing crawling on my stomach, using my arms to pull my body along. Then I used my legs to push forward without lifting my hips. The first obstacle was to swim across a lake and I was a weak swimmer, so I set about taking some swimming lessons.

My gym work turned to more functional training to build endurance, as well as good muscular strength and stamina. I went to a few sessions at the nearest CrossFit gym to work with more emphasis on timing and repetitious moves.

I could rejoice in the fact that I had been making war on my diseases and I was winning. My heart rate had improved so that I no longer needed to use an inhaler. My blood pressure was great in spite of my heart valves. I just really needed to keep the knees in good shape.

The question was how to prepare for this task mentally and emotionally. I would be on my own as I tackled each obstacle. The cheering squad was only in my head. Once we headed up the mountain, no one would be able to see us until we came to the last three obstacles—leaping three rows of fire, crawling under barbed wire, and getting through the last mud pit.

Everything between the first four obstacles and the last three was pure speculation. Information on-line only gave the planned obstacles, but nothing was certain except the run around the lake, the swim across the lake, a beach crawl through sand under barbed wire, and a rope climb up the fifteen-foot vertical wall. No problem, right?

What was so different about this and the other battles I had been in throughout my life? Combat between two elements is simple, right? Well, not quite. All parents have warred with their children from time to time. There are plenty of obstacles there.

Our bodies war with disease and changes of biological aging. Seen and unseen changes are happening all the time.

We all do battle in our own time and in our own way. When we run a race, we are aware of the start and finish line. In life, we do not have such clear markers in our struggles. Heart attacks do not always give you a warning. If you are not taking inventory, you would not know the possibility of one approaching. Sometimes, we battle for months or years before we can identify progress in our battles.

Mental struggles take a toll on us just as physical obstacles do. Children, jobs, school, and aging parents are all challenges we face in life.

My ongoing struggle is to perform every day at the best level of health possible. Yes, I have new struggles now—chemical allergies, both ingested and inhaled, which cause pulmonary issues. I like to breathe so I am forced to acknowledge some restrictions.

What if there was a better way to know our progress?

Is there a way to feel that we can achieve without being called a warrior?

Why do we so often have the mindset of "fighting a losing battle?"

This warrior knows that believing in yourself, being your own cheering squad, pushing through when the devil on your shoulder says, "give up," and accepting that sometimes it is necessary to fall back and regroup, are all parts of the character it takes to wage war. We wage war for what we believe to be true, right, and just. We wage war because we believe it will make us a better person in one way or another.

I am a warrior against all things that make me less than what I know I can do and be. My body has limitations but it also has had improvements and will continue to have improvements. I will war against the natural course of aging. There is no reason to give up— only reasons to continue on.

OBSTACLES ARE THOSE FRIGHTFUL THINGS YOU SEE
WHEN YOU TAKE YOUR EYES OFF THE GOAL.
— HENRY FORD

The time for the Warrior Dash had arrived. In May 2012, making the best preparations I knew how, I traveled to Mountain City, Georgia, checked into the motel room, and began to face all my doubts and fears. I drove up to the site of the race attempting to calm my emotions. I was ready to deal with the unknown challenges to come. Only the first few and last few obstacles were visible.

As the sun began to set, I made my way back to the motel, stopping to pick up some dinner. When I sat down to eat, doubt gripped me, making it difficult to swallow. Anxiety reached down deep into my soul, magnifying my doubts. Calming myself, I decided to go to bed and get a good night's sleep. Surely it would all look better in the morning.

I rose early the next day, went to get some breakfast, and returned to the motel. As I sat on the edge of the bed, I began to pray as earnestly as I had ever prayed in my life. "Lord, I know you have meant for me to do this. I am an old woman. I have accomplished a great deal so far, but this is really tough. If you want me to do this, I ask for your strength and your wisdom to handle each of the challenges in the race." This was going to be a real life-changing event.

When asked how long I thought the race would take me to finish, my best guess was about an hour. There was absolutely no basis for this answer, as it depended upon my belief in my ability.

At about 8 a.m. I made my way up to the site, found a parking place close by (with a water hose to wash off the mud) and began the check-in process. Later, I found Doc and he helped me tape up my knees. He took his place near the front of the line and I found myself standing between two girls wearing pink tutus. I felt so out of place, listening to the conversations of young, thin, bubbling guys and gals. It was like being in a nightmare.

Suddenly the horn blew, smoke and fire rose from the start line tower as barbaric cries filled the air and the crowd started moving. There was no turning back now. Put up or shut up time had arrived.

We all took the first quarter mile at a jog. As the group began to expand, I found myself passing a few people. Then I was behind two girls wearing shirts that said, YOU HAVE JUST BEEN PASSED BY A GIRL. I shifted my foot speed, passed the girls and said, "You've just been passed by a Grandma." Boy, did that feel great! Deep inside I knew it probably would not last.

Making my way to the lake, I caught a glance of runners already in the water, trying to gauge the best path to take. Unfortunately, it had rained heavily that week, so the lake was full to the banks. Moving to the right, I made my way in. The water was cold and dark. I moved with purpose, as fast as I could.

Suddenly my foot went down and my body dropped into the deep water. I raised my head up above the water, gasped for air, calmed myself, and began to swim for my life. I determined to keep my eye on the shore. Someone bumped me and I went under again but came up not quite as frightened as before. Stroking purposefully to stay calm and reach the shore was the only thought in my mind. Then, my feet felt the bottom and I breathed a sigh of relief.

Coming out on the shore, runners were presented with a course sand bed covered with barbed wire. I began to crawl, keeping the feet of the person in front of me in sight. I kept my head down, my body hugging the ground. Leg then arm, then leg and arm—I moved rhythmically. The width allowed only one carefully-moving person at a time. Then the height of the barbed wire rose about twelve inches higher, so I progressed quickly to the end of the obstacle.

We then moved freely down the road to the next unknown obstacle. There was a series of about six fences, each approximately five feet tall and six feet across, spaced three feet apart. I paused for a moment to watch someone else start the maneuver; over and under, over and under. Because the fence was almost as tall as I was, it was necessary to hoist my body up, fall to the ground, and slide under the next fence. I repeated the moves, rising up on my toes, throwing my legs over, breaking my fall as I hit the ground, and making the slide under the next fence. With each forward thrust of my leg over the fence top and each thump to the ground to crawl on the ground my shins lost one more layer of skin. My feet and clothes were soaking wet and covered in coarse sand. What a mess!

As we moved toward the next obstacle, my heart sank. Standing tall, in all its majesty, was the actualization of my fears. I thought, "I can do this. I can do this. I CAN DO THIS." But could I? This was the big one that frightened me the most.

When unsure of how to move, watch the other runners. Moving to the side for a few seconds, observing both men and women make the climb, I slowly approached the wall. It was a straight vertical wall, fifteen feet high. The ropes hung at intervals to provide room for arms and legs to move without hitting someone.

I grabbed the rope and positioned my hands for a good grip, but the sand made it difficult. On the first two tries the sand beneath my feet caused me to slide back down. Then I began to make my way up. When I reached the top, I placed my body on the top ridge and began to bring my legs over. One leg was up, but then the other leg lost its position, and I felt my body move.

My hands came off the wall. I reached out to grasp the rope. It was covered with slick black tape. My wet gloves could not get a safe grip and my body began to move back over the wall. In my mind, I could visualize what was happening. How could I stop it?

I was falling fast but I held tightly to the rope, hoping to make a good landing. Hope had left the scene and gone somewhere else. I hit the ground with both feet folded behind me and with my full body weight bearing down on them. The pain in my feet was at twenty on a scale of one to ten. Gathering my wits as those around me kindly inquired if I needed help, I rose and moved ever so slowly to the side of the trail and sat next to a race monitor. I was no stranger to pain and if there was one thing I had learned to deal with it was this pain.

The race monitor offered to take me to the first aid tent but I declined, quietly assessed my abilities, rose, and moved on.

The next obstacle was a dive into the water to an island in the small lake. Then we had to jump back in the water and swim the short distance to the shore. The obstacles continued. We climbed a cargo net; up one side and down the other. We climbed up a ladder, then across a cargo net, then down another ladder, then began a trek up the hill to the top of the mountain. Many asked if they could assist me as they went on their way. I thanked them all and was overwhelmed by their compassion. I knew that helping me would jeopardize their competition time. I continued on the narrow, slippery path in the woods.

As I approached the downhill side of the mountain I spotted a monitor. As I came closer he saw that I was limping. Again I was offered a ride to the first aid station. Again I declined. I asked for his first aid packet. He had some tape; I used it to tape my right ankle for better support. By now it was severely swollen and I dared not take off my shoe or loosen the strap. The best thing was to just keep moving.

I stepped back to the trail and tried to stay out of the way of passing runners. I encountered a slippery steep step on the trail. A young man offered help and would not move until he helped me on my way. I thanked him many times, knowing that he lost time while helping me.

The next obstacles were a fireman's pole, another cargo net climb, a downhill water slide, and then the end was in sight. A large area of tires required careful steps through rusty old vehicles. There was a short walk before the dreaded leap over fire, so I began to calculate how I could leap with a broken ankle. (Yes, I knew the ankle was broken, but I knew I would make it through.)

I had learned to run on my toes (instead of flat-footed) to help take stress off my knees, so I considered this my best option. I rose up on my toes, found the lowest pressure points on the right foot, and gave it a try. It worked. As I came closer to the fire and smoke, I could see there were three rows of fire. It was all or nothing at this point. Sure thing, Grandma. Easy as falling off a wall.

I took a long breath, never missed a step, and I began to run. I ran like I had never run in my life. Then I was over the first line, over the second line, and finally, over the third line headed for more barbed wire and the mud pit.

Through the mud pit, I raised my feet and walked on my hands. There is nothing like the feel of mud moving through your unmentionables. It gets into every crevice it can find.

At the end of the pit was the triumphant walk out to receive the coveted medal. My time was one hour, ten minutes. Not bad for a grandma with a broken ankle.

I waged war with my demons that day and I won. Although I struggled at times, there was never a doubt in my mind that God had brought me to that point to learn the power that has been given me. The power that says you can do anything you set your mind to do. The power that comes with challenges from all sides of life. With this power came the responsibility to teach others that they, too, have the same power.

I am a warrior against all those things that make me less than what I know I can do and be. There is no reason to give up. There are only reasons to continue on.

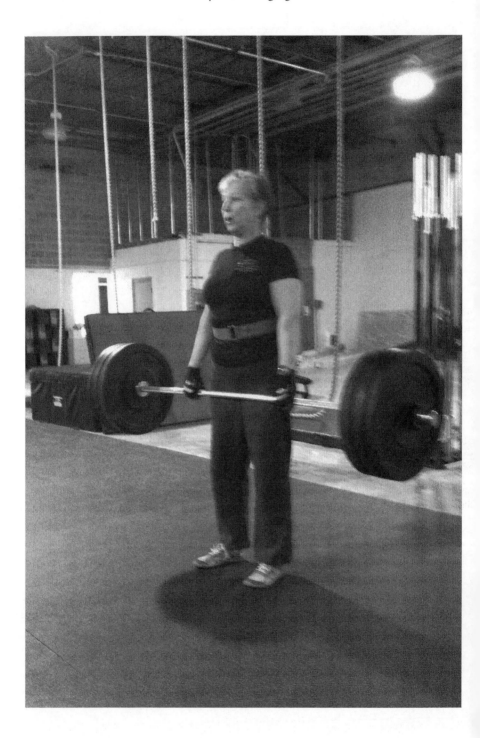

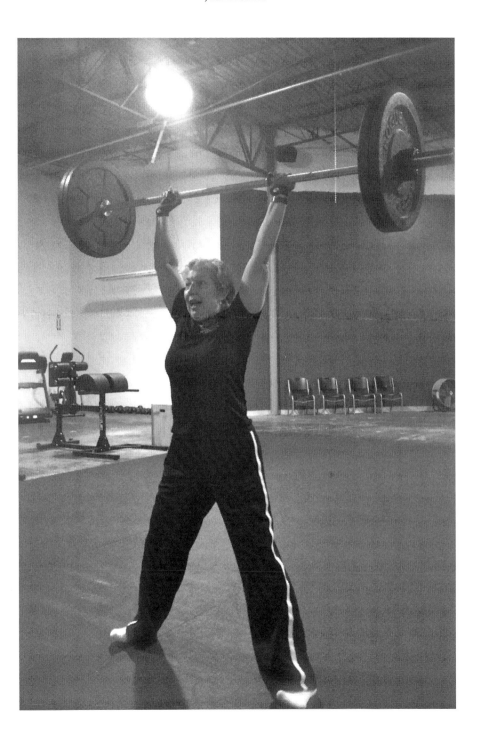

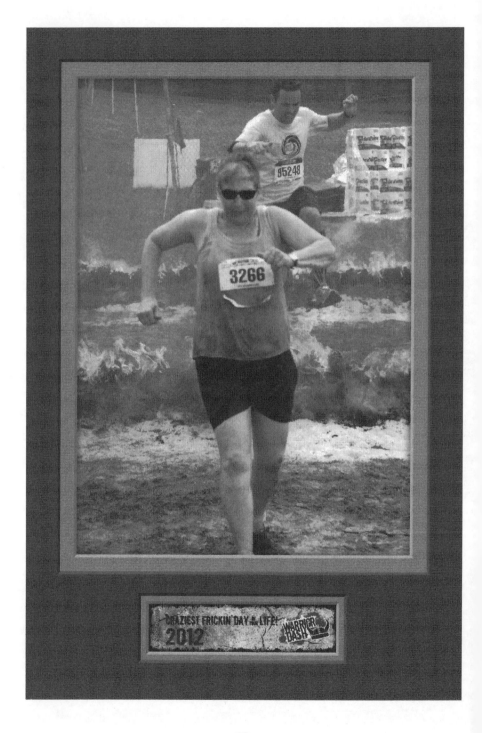

Chapter 6
DAY BY DAY

Progress lies not in enhancing what is, but in
advancing what will be.
— Khalil Gibran

Each day is a new opportunity to learn and grow, smell the roses, and share with others.

My adventures in exercise have taken me to yoga classes with an excellent instructor who taught me to breathe with movement, guiding my body in ways of less stress. Yoga with a broken ankle is a challenge, but it can be done. Learning to quiet the soul, control the mind, and move the body in synchrony is a beautiful thing.

As I carried my yoga training with me to the gym, the breathing lessons helped immensely as the weight training increased. When new challenges were offered, I accepted them in a new and clearer state of mind. That does not mean I was not challenged. It just means that my mind was clearer when approaching how to achieve them.

When frustrated or tired I took a few steps back, saw a chalkboard in my mind, then erased everything there. I could hear Doc's voice telling me the moves and I visualized them in my mind. As I stepped back up my inhale turned into an exhale and my body began to lift, press, push, or pull as needed. Each breath came at the time the body moved.

Calming the mind and spirit will help us to focus better on any issue we face, whether it is in the gym, the office, in traffic, or at home.

Next, my friend started a class in Pilates. Moves like "rolling like a ball" challenged me for months. My body had difficult visualizing itself in a "ball" when I knew that was impossible. Then one day as I kept telling myself not to lead with my shoulders, the tension left and there I went, rolling like a ball.

There are some moves that I have not yet accomplished, like standing on my head. But there are also new Pilates moves that I am doing.

Pilates is more appealing to me than yoga but they both should be in everyone's exercise list. The reduced joint impact is a primary feature of Pilates while gaining strength and flexibility. Core strengthening is in every movement. Because of this, I became a Pilates instructor.

Pilates has moves for everyone at every age and every level of fitness. Recently a Facebook post featured Sylvester Stallone on the Pilates reformer at age 70. Pilates has recently been credited for helping professional athletes in baseball and football. Truly it is for everyone.

Joseph Pilates, a chiropractor, created the original Pilates regimen while treating soldiers after the war. His studio in New York was next door to a ballet studio and the dancers soon became clients to help keep fit and recover from injuries.

Each day, each new client, each new mental and physical challenge is an opportunity to learn and grow. Why would we not want that in our lives? Why would I decide to not live to a fuller and higher level?

Chronological age and physical age do not have to be the same. We can turn the clock back on physical aging if we are truly ready to accept the challenge.

I now see my ability to live alone from a different perspective. These experiences challenged me to learn more about the anatomy of my feet and how they impact movement. In 2016 I became a Certified Barefoot Training Specialist. This was an eye-opening study that emphasized just how lucky I had been in my recovery each time. This study has shown how little the public really knows about the importance of our feet. When our feet hurt, everything hurts. When we have injuries, the body compensates in ways you might never expect. Pain is our only clue, and it is up to us to find the cause and correct it.

As we become aware of the challenges of aging, we can accept the challenge to hold those challenges back, before they become a problem to deal with. If I only knew then what I know now, my fifties would have been so much better.

If we have to change, why not change for the better?

I have recovered from broken ankles, torn muscles and ligaments in both my feet and bunion surgery. These were all opportunities to broaden my anatomical knowledge and learn to understand mobility challenges.

We should all be open to learning about the way our bodies move. It is life changing knowledge. Become aware of what you don't know.

Chapter 7
IT'S ALL IN YOUR HEAD

I am seeking. I am striving. I am in it with all my heart.
— Van Gogh

The hard question is, "Are you content to remain broken?"

When did it become acceptable to bankrupt our physical health?

Your past need not become your future.

Have you ever stood in front of the mirror and conversed with yourself about the pros and cons of doing something? Did you visualize the angel on one shoulder and the devil on the other shoulder? Were you honest in all your thoughts?

Not all of our thoughts are true. Who would dare say such a thing! The mental debate that sometimes rages in our head can be calmed and controlled. This I came to learn.

Our brain is an absolute wonder. It contains electricity. It contains drugs. It contains traffic signals for messaging.

Just as our cars and trucks require routine maintenance, so does our brain. Each night when we go to bed there is a routine that the brain is performing not too unlike charging your cellphone battery. Our body has to have time to recharge and repair. Without restorative sleep we begin to have failure in our system messaging and our bodies cannot function at the normal processing rate.

You depend on your car for transportation to get you where you want and need to go. Each time you get behind the wheel you expect that engine to start. Your body is no less important. It requires the right fuel to perform. It requires the right mixture of food and rest to regenerate. When it doesn't get the right combination of nutrition, rest and recovery time it won't work correctly. Your car won't run if you don't put the fuel and oil and air in the tires regularly.

Excuses and reasons are not the same things. Excuses are parts of us that want to remain comfortable and content—broken. Humanity finds excuses for remaining broken every day.

The mental challenges can be met. Is it easy? Nothing in life is free or easy. You have to put in the work. You have to accept the mental challenges as well as the physical challenges.

In one year I was able to stop taking medication for asthma, high cholesterol, high blood pressure, depression, and anxiety. I was able to come out of chronic pain. To this day I do not have chronic pain.

My left knee required surgery in 2013, which broke my heart and caused me anguish. I had lots of conversation with myself about how to recover, how long it would take to recover and questioned if I would lose all that I had worked so hard to gain. Deep inside, though, I knew it was necessary. My recovery took eighteen long months to bring me back to doing squats and lifting weights.

My best lift was a two-hundred-pound dead lift. Never would I have attempted it without the training and encouragement from my friend, Todd. We all want someone in our corner cheering us on, telling us we can do what we really don't believe we can. In real life, we do not always have a cheering gallery when we want one so we must learn to use the power and strength we have been given.

So how do we keep that motivation when there is no cheering squad?

Keep having those conversations with yourself while you are taking walks or cooking. Positive conversations with yourself are fine if they are positive and really truthful. Once you get your mind in the ditch it is so easy to stay there but in reality *we must not stay there.*

Have you ever heard of neuroplasticity or mental imagery?

Yes, it is all in your head. Literally and figuratively it is all in your head. Your marvelous brain works with your thoughts whether they are positive or negative. Whether you WANT to do something or just say you want to is all in your head.

Neuroplasticity is the ability to redirect your brain waves and change your thoughts. I am not surprised if you have not heard of it. There is a very clear mind-body connection and we hear the term mind-body more now than in the past. Our fast paced world makes it difficult to stop and take a moment to "reboot" our system but it is so very crucial for our mind and our body to take that time.

Numerical aging will happen and it really can be a good thing to reach 40 or 50 instead of lingering on the 'concept' of being OLD. There is so much in the world to see and do and so much of ourselves to just be and live. But you cannot maintain youth if you don't take care of yourself both mentally and physically. Change those brainwave patterns and change both your outlook and your physical ability.

Mental imagery for me began in the early 1990's after my husband left me and our two children after 15 years of marriage. As many who have been in this path learned, we are not prepared for that. Fortunately for me, I was introduced to mental imagery to treat depression and anxiety. That was quite a lesson.

We all have times that we just can't seem to clear the clutter in our minds. Work, school, children, soccer, scouts, grocery shopping, car to the shop for an oil change. It just never seems to stop. And of course, there are other issues that crowd in when role reversal takes place with our parents or grandparents.

Remember, the mind dictates to the body, not the reverse. Stop and breathe, clear your mind. Remove everything from between your ears. Put a blank chalkboard up there and simply write on it what you need/want your body to do.

Living alone and maintaining independence as we age can be very challenging. Doing everything you can to remain self-sufficient is a must. Exercise can be simple. Working with bands and balls with proper training in proper form can work wonders to keep us fit for simple daily tasks.

This is not a guilt trip. This is a warning. We are responsible for the care and upkeep of our mental, emotional, and physical abilities. Be a good steward of what you have been given. Start early before the aging process gets a grip on you.

Chapter 8
GOOD NUTRITION

*Your body keeps an accurate record of what you
put in it whether you do or not.*
— Unknown

DIET is a four letter word that simply means Did I Eat Today.

Much is said about having a good diet or a bad diet. I propose we change that to good nutrition or poor nutrition. Nutrition is what you give your body to keep it going smoothly and at capacity.

Do you know someone who struggles with a continuous cycle of weight gain and weight loss? Do you know someone who is tired all the time?

Body chemistry is not the same every day and no two people have the exact same body chemistry. Our BMR, Basil Metabolic Rate, changes based on our activity OR lack of activity. Thus, one size does not fit all and when it comes to fueling your body, time needs to be spent educating yourself on how your particular body metabolism is working.

When I began my physical training I thought I had a good diet but I did not know what I did not know. When I was diagnosed with high cholesterol the doctor gave me a pamphlet from the American Heart

Association and told me to change my diet. So I went with what the research of the time told me was best to NOT eat. The problem with that philosophy was that it only gave me a view from the cholesterol perspective, not the view of a full day's requirement of food. Of course research has changed since then.

The brochure gave me information about foods that were high in cholesterol and a few options for those. Some of my favorite things were banned: eggs, coconut, chocolate, and cheese to name a few. That was twenty-five years ago. At that time food did not have all the chemicals that today's food contains. We know so much more about good fats and bad fats.

Our markets contain foods from many more countries than were available twenty-five years ago. Remember that everything you eat and drink is filtered through your liver. That means every aspirin or Tylenol, or prescription medication, or gin and tonic, or beer is filtered for properties that belong and can be used by your body. If you take statin medications did you ever ask why the doctor takes blood tests every three months? They are checking your liver function. Think about it. Liver failure is not a good thing.

Our bodies require good nutrition to function optimally. Carbohydrates, fats, and proteins in proper balance will keep your body running like a finely tuned car. The carbohydrates are fuel, the fats are the oil to mix with the fuel, and the protein maintains our muscle structure that holds our bones together. Hydration to keep our body fluids moving is critical.

Carbohydrates, such as bread and white potatoes, are processed and used quite differently than carbohydrates from Romaine lettuce, beets, broccoli, or spinach. Nuts and seeds have good fats as do avocados and olive oil. Nuts, seeds, and leafy greens are just a few of the foods that also provide much-needed fiber in our diet.

If you have ever eaten your favorite food cooked fresh with all natural ingredients, then compared it to the same food that came prepackaged in the store, you would find a number of "added" ingredients that are not natural. Our bodies were not made to process these chemicals.

Let's look at a very common food that is given to our children without a second thought—M&Ms. The ingredient list looks like this: milk chocolate (sugar, chocolate, skim milk, cocoa butter, lactose, milk fat, soy lecithin, salt, artificial flavors, sugar, cornstarch, less than 1% corn syrup, dextrin, coloring (includes Blue 1 Lake, Red 40, Yellow 6, Yellow 5, Blue 1, Red 40 Lake, Yellow 5 Lake, Yellow 6 Lake, Blue 2 Lake, Blue 2, Gum Acacia. One serving of fifteen pieces has eight grams of fat (five grams saturated fat), twenty-nine grams of carbohydrates (twenty-six of those grams are sugar), and two grams of protein. The caloric count for these fifteen pieces is two hundred. *Consider that the twenty-six grams of sugar come from straight granulated sugar, corn syrup, and cornstarch. That leaves three grams of carbohydrates to come from artificial food color, chocolate, and milk products. That makes only 3 grams of carbohydrates to use for fuel.*

So what happens when we eat these items? Putting it quite simply, the artificial ingredients are filtered through our liver. If they are not processed for nutritional value in our bodies, they are stored as fat.

Calories are not created equal. Learning about good natural food and being aware of what you are putting in your body is essential for good health. Poor nutrition equals poor body function.

Fad diets do not work because they do not take into consideration the individual lifestyle, the chronological age, or the activity of the individual. Good nutrition must become a matter of lifestyle.

It took me almost two years to find the right combination of food that my body needed and used. Don't settle for the same old rhetoric from the medical community, "eat a good diet and exercise."

I struggled with my weight my entire life. Yes, there were family issues and yes, there were nutritional issues at times, but we had good wholesome food on the table three meals a day based on the knowledge available at the time. Oleomargarine is terrible for us but we did not know it back then. Bread is not needed at every meal. Dessert is not needed at every meal and was certainly not intended as our breakfast. Carbonated beverages are full of sugar but in my teens, they were just making the scene.

All of my clients who tell me they want to lose weight get the same message from me. You must adjust your nutritional food intake and you must exercise to build muscle. Muscle burns more calories than fat. Use the stored fat to fuel your body.

Your food intake does not need to be complicated. You just need to learn what you are eating and why you need to eat it. On several occasions, I have spoken to groups about nutrition. The response has been a jaw dropping, "I didn't know that." My favorite two shockers are; (1) a serving size is usually one-half cup and (2) the baked beans you are eating from a can contains fifty percent sugar. Then comes the question from me, "Will this change your eating habits?"

For those with inflammation here are a list of the top 15 anti-inflammatory foods:

1. Green leafy vegetables. These are rich in antioxidants.

2. Bok Choy

3. Celery

4. Beets -These are full of folate, manganese, potassium and magnesium.

5. Broccoli

6. Blueberries

7. Pineapple

8. Salmon

9. Bone Broth

10. Walnuts

11. Coconut Oil

12. Chia Seeds

13. Flaxseeds

14. Turmeric

15. Ginger

These are readily available in grocery stores.

Protein is a subject near and dear to me. As we age we continue to lose muscle fiber. Between the ages of 20 and 70 the average loss of muscle is 40%. Did I hear some jaws dropping? That is a loss of about 8% muscle fiber per decade; or about 1% loss per year.

So let's look at this another way. If a 40 year old weighs 160 pounds and their body is 40% muscle and 60% fat, generally active about twice a week (weekends), and are not taking action to restore muscle nutritionally and physically, by the time they are age 50 approximately 8%-10% more muscle will be lost.

If this pattern continues bone density decreases, shoulders and lower back aches and pains become more prevalent, activity decreases, posture suffers and falls become more likely. No one wants to go there but some are well on their way.

According to the 2015-2020 U.S. Dietary Guidelines for Americans, "Today, about half of all American adults—117 million people—have one or more preventable, chronic diseases, many of which are related to poor quality eating patterns and physical inactivity. Rates of these chronic, diet-related diseases continue to rise, and they come not only with increased health risks, but also at high cost."

Specific charts in this report reflect our intake of carbohydrates to be above the recommended levels and our intake of proteins to be below the recommended levels.

This year the life expectancy in the United States for both men and women dropped.

These are my personal recommendations for everyone:

1. Try not to eat any prepared foods that have more than 5 ingredients on the label.

2. Always compare the nutritional value on the packages with the contents. Example: How many of the carbohydrates are sugars and how much of the fat is saturated? Is it a good source for fiber and protein?

3. The main ingredient in the product should be listed first. The law requires food labels to list ingredients in the order of their respective amounts. Example: The M&M package said the main ingredient was milk chocolate, with sugar and cornstarch listed next.

4. Vegetables and produce should be purchased in season whenever possible to provide the maximum amount of nutritional value. Fresh produce can be prepared at home quickly, and just as easily, as canned. Baked vegetables, such as asparagus, carrots, beets, and squash—especially fall and winter squash—taste delicious and are great as leftovers in soups and stews.

5. Our modern bodies were not made to digest gluten. Eat as little gluten as possible.

6. Eat only non-GMO products.

7. Drink water, water, and more water.

Eat Well. Think Positive. Move Often.

Chapter 9
FUNCTIONAL TRAINING

Believe you can and you are halfway there.
— Theodore Roosevelt

Americans spend billions of dollars each year on exercise and weight loss programs. In my personal opinion, the most important exercise program you can do is Functional Training.

Take a moment to consider your health and fitness level right now.

What do you have difficulty doing: climbing stairs, walking for extended periods of time, putting boxes up on the closet shelf, vacuuming the floors, taking out the trash, getting in and out of the car? Those things are activities of daily living (ADL).

What do you want to be able to do *now*? What is on your bucket list?

My experiences in the fitness industry, perspectives from my training, and feedback from my clients; these have given me a world of knowledge most gym trainers do not have. I have physically done and studied standard personal trainer philosophy through my certification as a personal trainer with the American Council on Exercise (ACE). I have also studied, and I teach, Pilates. During the four years since my study with ACE began, I have completed many courses on working with older adults and individuals with challenges from diabetes, cardiopulmonary disease, and arthritis. My studies in 2016 were focused on the foot and the roles it plays in our ability to stand and move. This was done through the Evidence Based Fitness Academy. My clients currently range from fifty to eighty-five and they all have unique issues to deal with. One exercise theory fits them all—Functional Training.

Mayo Clinic's electronic newsletter describes functional fitness as exercises that train your muscles to work together and prepare them for daily tasks by simulating common movements you might do at home, at work, or in sports. While using various muscles in the upper and lower body at the same time, functional fitness exercises also emphasize core stability.

Please read that one more time and think about every move you made from the time you got out of bed this morning.

Functional training is for movement. Our bodies were made to move and are constructed so intricately with the grace and majesty of a fifty-story architectural marvel. Everything is connected and working together to do the smallest tasks.

Moving from side to side, up and down, to the front and to the back takes coordination of a multitude of muscles, tendons and ligaments, and joints.

CrossFit™, which is based upon functional training describes it as "Universal motor recruitment patterns; [which] are performed in a wave of contraction from core to extremity; and [which] are compound movements; i.e. they are multi-joint."

A client once asked me, "What muscle am I using when I do this?" No one muscle moves in isolation. For each contraction of muscle there is an opposite extension. Muscles work in groups to accomplish our body's movement.

Functional Training Includes Ten Elements: Cardio and Respiratory Endurance, Stamina, Strength, Flexibility, Power, Speed, Coordination, Agility, and Balance. What is your current exercise regimen? Does it include all of these within a week's timeframe?

Individuals may be trained on these elements at their own unique level. When I started my training, I knew nothing of "functional" elements of exercise or how they related to my daily tasks. What I have learned from my clients and audiences is that we, as a people, do not know how to care for ourselves nor do we understand how our bodies move. For those presently 40 and older there is no better time like the present to begin your training.

To become a Pilates instructor, it is required to study body movement, also called kinesiology. Studying to be a certified personal trainer does not usually go into the depth of each muscle and joint as required by Pilates. Pilates also grades students on observed student teaching and with both an oral and written exam.

Only one of my clients has a working knowledge of the body. She is a retired nurse. My younger clients who are working professionals were not taught the information needed to understand their body. With a gym on every corner, the education continues to be nonexistent. I was lucky—curiosity put me with the right teacher and helping my mother study during her nurse training gave me some basis for my curiosity of medical conditions.

Is it any wonder the nation is having an obesity epidemic, that arthritis pain is the number one cause of work absences, and medical insurance is so expensive? Drug companies are making millions from our ignorance.

Take responsibility for your life, your ability to live *your* way, and the way to prevent aging before aging prevents you from a full life.

Chapter 10
WHAT IF?

Our greatest glory is not in never failing, but in
rising up every time we fail.
— Ralph Waldo Emerson

We make decisions every day, all during the day. Having a problem and choosing to do nothing is making a decision.

What if you always thought you hated exercise but learned that not all exercise is done in a gym? Exercise is moving your body in a specific way to use specific muscles. That does not sound so complicated.

What if there were ways to do functional exercise in every day for ten to fifteen minutes? Would you do it?

What if exercising meant that you could go up and down stairs with ease?

What if it meant you could pick up objects without fear of hurting your back or falling down?

Be honest with yourself. What do you have to lose by trying?

What do you have to lose by facing your pain and fears in order to gain strength and energy for everyday living?

What if you could hold your grandchildren, play with them, share your life with them just by changing your mindset about exercise?

What if you took a few minutes to research personal trainers to find one near you to help you meet your goals?

What if you actually found someone who would be happy to work with you, as you are now, teach you how to be better and do more?

We cannot all be perfect physical specimens. Some of us must be more diligent than others. Some of us are just content to be unhappy, unhealthy and aging faster than others.

No, I, for one, will not go quietly. I will be thankful to rise up each morning. I will be thankful that I can function well and not worry about falling.

I will dance like no one is watching. I will lift my weights for strong bones. I will savor the ability to go up and down my basement stairs to do laundry.

What if you could be better than you are today?

Create your own reality. Start today.

Be Brave. Be in Control. Be Powerful.

CLIENT TESTIMONIALS

"I have had several personal trainers over the years but not one of them can hold a candle to Nancy. Nancy is unique and every training session is different and tailored to accommodate her clients' needs and capabilities. She teaches you how to do the exercise with proper form. If you ever have the opportunity to train with her, you will not be disappointed."

- NICOLE MAC

"At 64 I wish I had been doing this a lifetime but if not a lifetime at least the last decade because there is power in being able to control where your body goes."

- PAMELA

"I think too many people have been told getting old is the end of the road. And I accepted that for a while and I was bed-ridden, I weighed 94 pounds, I was starving to death. I didn't move, I couldn't walk. I had to use a walker. I started exercising. I started going to water aerobics, but Nancy has made such a difference in my life."

- SHERRY

"No one wants to age and watch as our bodies slowly deteriorate with age related issues we take for granted are not preventable. But they are preventable! I started training with Nancy and through her instruction and workout regime, now understand how important a

program devoted to strengthening my core and every bone and muscle in my body is to thwarting aging and staying healthy. Understanding and adopting this philosophy has been a life changing experience for me and will be for you!"

- KATHY

About the Author

Nancy K. Burnham is the owner of Simple Fitness LLC in Lilburn, Georgia. As a Successful Aging Specialist, her objective is to help individuals have a healthier and happier tenure while they are Moving Through Life™. She began her return to health in 2008 when she walked into a local gym and hired a personal trainer. Within a year she was no longer taking five prescription medications. At the age of sixty-four, while still under the tutelage of her personal trainer, she recognized that older adults—people like her—were not receiving the same level of training because the younger trainers did not know how to work with the older members. As a result, she began her studies to become a certified personal trainer through the American Council on Exercise. While in the gym the older members would tell her how encouraging she was to them.

In July 2012, Nancy became certified as a trainer, having passed the exam, and immediately proceeded to study additional information regarding older "special" populations. At that time there were no certifications available for training older adults. She took courses in cardiovascular disease, diabetes, shoulder injuries, knee problems, and lumbo-pelvic stabilization.

Nancy's philosophy as a personal trainer became clear when she read an article in the Idea Fitness Journal (September 2012) by Len Kravitz, PhD.

"A great personal trainer empowers clients to believe they truly are in control of their health and well-being. These trainers have a stirring faith in their clients' individual abilities and they help people relax and believe in themselves. Great trainers don't teach personal training—they teach each client."

In 2013 she attended CrossFit™ training and later that same year received a certificate in Pilates training. She also holds certificates as a Fitness Coaching Specialist, a Senior Fitness Specialist, Total Barre™ instructor, and ZenGA™ instructor.

In 2016, she became a Certified Barefoot Training Specialist Level 1, foot to core sequencing and foot anatomy. She also attended Barefoot Training Specialist Level 2 which relates to issues arising from improper gait.

She has been featured in the Atlanta-Journal Constitution newspaper and the Living Better 50 online magazine and referenced in Energy Times magazine.

Nancy has spoken at the local senior center on several occasions and provided free class instruction on nutrition and exercise. She has also made presentations to weight loss groups and a networking organization.

She can be contacted at 770-289-8883 or nancyssimplefitness@gmail.com regarding speaking engagements, nutrition or fitness matters.

FREE OFFER

Visit my website today to schedule your
free 1-Hour consultation.

NancyKBurnham.com

My home studio is quiet and private. There is
no embarrassment about ability or question too
inconsequential to be discussed.

My training sessions are private to meet each
client's specific goals and needs mutually agreed
upon before beginning a plan.

Session Packages are available for

4,6 and 8 Week Programs @ 2 sessions a week

USE CODE Book 1
FOR 10% DISCOUNT

I offer small classes for mat Pilates in
groups of 2 – 4 people.

I am also available to meet with your business staff,
EAP, civic organization, or club with directed or
general exercise and nutritional information.

My newsletter is available on line.

Please feel free to send any comments or questions
to me at **nancyssimplefitness@gmail.com**